TABLE OF CONTENT.

1.

INTRODUCTION.

Being fat is a complicated illness that involves redundant body fat. Being fat is further than simply a visual issue. It's a medical condition that raises the possibility of multitudinous other ails and health issues. Heart affections, hypertension, high cholesterol situations, diabetes, liver complaint, sleep apnea, and some types of cancer is an exemplifications of these. There are multitudinous explanations for why some people struggle with weight loss. rotundity is constantly caused by heritable, physiological, and environmental variables, in addition to choices made about nutrition, exercise, and physical exertion. The positive aspect is that rotundity- related health issues can be avoided or bettered with indeed a small quantum of weight loss. You can reduce your weight by espousing new actions, eating a healthier diet, and exercising further. Other choices for managing rotundity include traditional specifics and weight- loss ways.

CHAPTER ONE; A LOOK INTO THE OBESITY EPIDEMIC.

Originally, let us get familiar with the obesity epidemic.

For both adults and children, obesity raises the risk of numerous chronic diseases. Over time, the obesity epidemic seems to have started with a small but steady positive energy balance.

Although there isn't enough data to conclude that obesity has been successfully addressed, significant public health initiatives are being made in this area. Obesity is probably one of the most challenging public health concerns our society has ever encountered because of its complexity.

Numerous ailments, including diabetes, cardiovascular disease, and cancer, are more common in those who are obese.

When paired with other parameters like waist circumference, the body mass index (BMI) can be a useful tool for predicting negative cardiovascular outcomes. However, its predictive power is limited when used alone.

The knowledge gathered from past epidemiologic issues, like smoking, should assist those concerned in expanding necessary health programs and raising the possibility that future generations won't face the negative effects of obesity.

The commercial sector, non-governmental organizations, civil society, governments, and foreign partners all have important responsibilities to play in the fight against obesity.

For the far too many obese adults and children, we need to know more about how to stop or slow the onset of obesity-related illnesses and disabilities.

Despite body mass index's lack of sensitivity to variations in body composition or body fat distribution, at the population level, we can likely detect the health hazards associated with obesity on its own.

However, a much more sophisticated approach is needed to comprehend the numerous and diverse mechanisms through which extra body fat may result in unfavorable health outcomes.

The scope and course of the obesity pandemic represent shifts in the cultures in which we live and present a challenge to us in figuring out changeable avenues that will have enough effect to stop the epidemic for everyone.

CHAPTER TWO: CAUSES AND

SYMPTOMS OF OBESITY

Generally speaking, the following factors increase the risk of weight gain: fast food, Fried foods, such as french fries, treated and fatty meats, dairy products in excess, baked goods with added sugar, prepared breakfast cereals, and a variety of other packaged and packaged foods that include added refined sugar, drinks such as soda, smoothies with added sweeteners, and alcoholic beverages. Breads and bagels are among the many carbs found in manufactured meals.Though body weight is influenced by genes, habits, metabolism, and hormones, obesity is mostly caused by consumption of more calories than losing them during everyday tasks and physical exercise. Your body stores these excess calories as fat.Western workers now typically work in significantly less physically demanding jobs, which means they burn fewer calories there. Some of the symptoms that accompany obesity includes;

- panting for air.
- elevated perspiration.
- snores.
- trouble engaging in physical exercise.
- feeling exhausted all the time.
- back and joint aches.
- low self-esteem and confidence.

Panting for air;
Obesity hypoventilation syndrome is more likely to develop in those who

are overweight or obese. Sleep apnea is a common complication of obese hypoventilation syndrome.

The reason why some obese individuals experience obesity hypoventilation syndrome while others do not is unknown. Excess fat around your neck, chest, or belly might cause hormones that alter your body's breathing rhythms and make it harder for you to breathe deeply. It is possible that there is an issue with the way the human brain regulates your breathing.

Elevated perspiration;

Being overweight makes it difficult for the body to operate normally, which leads to a number of issues. Often, this results in excessive perspiration. Sweating is the result of the body temperature rising as a result of the heart pumping harder to pump oxygenated blood cells into the body.

Snores;

Fat deposits in the neck can narrow the upper airway, making it more difficult for you to breathe when you're lying down, which can lead to snoring. It can also occur when fat in your midsection area compresses your lungs and rib cage, collapsing your throat and making breathing harder.

Trouble engaging in physical exercise;

Obesity and Overweight Increase the Risk of Exercise-Related Injuries. This may hold true based on the degree of extra weight and the kinds of exercise. People who are overweight may be more vulnerable to accidents due to increased torque on their weight-bearing joints, particularly their knees and ankles.

Feeling exhausted all the time;

The relationship between obesity and chronic fatigue is influenced by multiple factors: Being obese raises your risk of developing sleep apnea, a condition that interferes with breathing and impairs sleep. Fatigue can be caused by insulin resistance, which is frequent in obese people and can progress to diabetes if ignored.

Back and joint aches;

Obesity has been linked to disk degeneration, sciatica, and lower back pain, among other forms of back pain. Being overweight strains your spine and may cause damage to the disks between your vertebrae. Your posture may also be impacted by carrying too much weight around your breasts and abdomen.

Low self-esteem and confidence;

Does Obesity Affect Self-Esteem? Research and clinical examinations have demonstrated that advanced obesity has a statistically significant effect on an individual's emotional, psychological, and physical fitness. Adult obesity is associated with sedentary behavior, emotional instability, and a decreased sense of self-assurance.

CHAPTER THREE; OBESITY FROM THE MEDICAL VIEW.

Body mass index, or BMI, is a commonly used diagnostic tool for obesity.Most people can use their BMI to fairly determine how much body fat they have. However, BMI does not directly assess body fat. Some people, such as physically active athletes, may be classified as obese by BMI if they do not have excessive body fat. Many medical professionals also consider an individual's waist circumference when deciding on a course of treatment. This measurement is known as your waist circumference. Males who measure their waists larger than forty-inch (102 cm) are prone to have health problems related to their weight. Women are prone to have these if their waist measurements are over thirty-five inches (89 cm). An additional statistic to track development.

Nowadays, obesity is the fifth-leading cause of mortality worldwide. Obesity and its related disorders have become serious health issues around the world. Uneven energy distribution between calories spent and calories ingested is the primary cause of obesity and overweight.

A straightforward index used to place humans into one of three categories— "underweight," "overweight," or "obese"—the "Body Mass Index" (BMI) is calculated as [(weight in kg)/(height in m2)." Despite being created in the 1830s by a sociologist and mathematician from Belgium, BMI is still frequently used to quantify obesity and obesity trends.

Numerous studies have shown that obesity is a complicated health issue resulting from a mixture of major causes (unhealthy society or cultural eating patterns, food deserts) and individual variables (genetics, learnt behaviors).

Additionally, studies have shown that obesity in all its forms, including abdominal obesity, is linked to a higher chance of developing a number of chronic illnesses and diseases, such as diabetes, cancer, asthma, hypercholesterolemia, and cardiovascular disorders.

Therefore, although obesity is definitely a medical condition, it also causes new conditions and aggravates those that already exist. Furthermore, a number of cardiovascular diseases (CVDs), including hypertension, coronary heart disease (CHD), atrial fibrillation (AF), and even complete heart failure, are becoming more common as a result of obesity.

Individuals' susceptibility to adult obesity is influenced by hereditary and lifestyle factors. Consequently, notable obesity clusters in particular geographic locations and situations also indicate the influence of socioeconomic as well as environmental elements in environments that are "obesogenic."

Due to the previously mentioned extra complexities, comprehending the causes and drivers of obesity is a key first step toward formulating successful policy and feasible preventative strategies.

Without a thorough understanding of the many connections between the various obesity risk factors and the science behind them, efforts will not be successful.

Despite the fact that a number of research have focused on obesity and overweight, systematic literature reviews (SLRs) along with comparable summaries that identify the factors that may contribute to and influence adult obesity are still required.

As a result, the causes of adult obesity and the state of the art and upcoming research in this area are methodically examined in this SLR.

Therefore, in order to suggest fresh, evidence-based strategies and remedies for adult obesity, this project will encourage collaborations between state-of-the-art research, medical expertise, and policy makers.

CHAPTER FOUR; PROBLEMS ASSOCIATED WITH OBESITY

Serious health diseases and challenges with daily tasks are only a couple of the additional issues that obesity can lead to.

Dyspnea,
Increased perspiration
Snoring,
Difficulties exercising,
Frequent fatigue,
Back and joint discomfort,
Low self-esteem,
A sense of isolation.

Obesity-related psychological issues can lead to depression and have an impact on your relationships with friends and family.

severe medical issues.
Additionally, obesity raises your chance of a number of potentially dangerous medical disorders, such as: Type 2 diabetes is a disorder that can result in excessive blood sugar.
high blood pressure,
high cholesterol, and atherosclerosis, or the narrowing of the arteries by fatty deposits.
These conditions can cause major heart disease and stroke.
An instant cure exists for obesity. Programs for losing weight need effort and dedication and are most effective when they are finished. The medical staff who are providing your care ought to offer support and guidance on how to keep off the weight you have lost.
It might also be beneficial to regularly check your weight, make reasonable objectives, and involve your loved ones in your weight loss efforts. Recall that even seemingly insignificant weight loss—3% or more of your starting body weight—can substantially lower your lifetime chance of acquiring diabetes and heart disease, two conditions linked to obesity.
elevated blood pressure Blood circulates through your blood arteries more forcefully than usual when you have NIH the outside link, also known as hypertension. Because your heart must work more tirelessly to pump blood to all of your cells, having an enormous physique might raise blood pressure. Your kidneys, which aid in controlling blood pressure, may be harmed by excess fat.a

CHAPTER FIVE; SOLVING THE OBESITY PUZZLE.

Eating a nutritious, low-calorie diet and getting regular exercise are the best ways to cure obesity. This is what you should do:

Consume a diet that is calorie-controlled and well-balanced, as advised by your physician or a weight-loss specialist (e.g., a dietitian).

Participate in 150–300 minutes (two and a half to five hours) of physical activity, such as brisk walking, running, swimming, or tennis, by joining a local losing weight program. a week.

Eat mindfully and stay away from circumstances where you might be tempted to overindulge.

Getting psychological treatment from a qualified healthcare provider may also be beneficial for you in order to alter your perspective on food and eating.

If modifying your lifestyle doesn't help you lose weight on its own, a prescription called orlistat might be suggested.

There are several strategies to avoid obesity in children and adults, despite the rising rates. We'll discuss both of these in this article, along with the progress made in reducing obesity.

Prevention of obesity starts early. It's critical to support youth in maintaining an ideal weight without putting too much emphasis on weight.

Childhood obesity risk was found to be lower in those who breastfed. The benefits of breastfeeding in preventing obesity have been the subject of conflicting research, thus further study is required.

Toddlers don't need a lot of food to thrive. For children aged 1 to 3, approximately 40 calories should be consumed for every inch of height. Encourage older kids to research the differences between serving sizes.

From a young age, encourage your child to sample a range of fruits, vegetables, and proteins. They could be more inclined to include these healthful foods in their own diet as they get older.

It is possible to introduce healthy eating to children at a young age by making dietary changes as a family. As they get older, it will be simpler for them to maintain their healthy eating practices.

If you eat though you're not hungry, you may end up overeating. Overconsumption of fuel can eventually result in obesity as it is stored as body fat. To improve digestion, teach your child to chew food more slowly and to only eat when they are truly hungry.

Your youngster may be more prone to eat unhealthy foods if you bring them into the home. Instead of keeping unhealthy snacks in the cupboard and refrigerator, try to keep healthier options on hand for occasional "treats."

Every day, children and teenagers should engage in at least 60 minutes of physical activityTrusted Source.

Engaging in games, sports, gym classes, or even outdoor chores are enjoyable physical activities. Less time for exercise and restful sleep is correlated with increased screen time. Exercise and sleep are more crucial for maintaining a healthy weight than screen time or television. Insufficient sleep can lead to increased weight in both adults and children (Trusted Source). According to the National Sleep Foundation, having a comfy pillow and mattress, a sleep regimen, and a nightly ritual are all examples of healthy sleep habits. Youngsters have lots of opportunity to eat unhealthy meals outside of the home, whether they are at institution of learning, with friends, or being watched. Though it's not always possible to watch over their diet, you can still be helpful by making inquiries. Many of these strategies for preventing obesity also apply to maintaining or reducing weight to a healthy level. In summary, maintaining a healthy weight can be prevented by increasing physical activity and consuming a balanced diet.
Obesity risk is correlated with nutrition and the use of ultra-processed and processed foods. Excessive consumption of processed foods can be promoted by their excessive sugar, salt, and fats content.
Adults should aim to consume between five and nine dishes of fruits and vegetables each day. Fruit and vegetables can help you keep your calorie intake in check and lower your chance of overindulging.

Feeling supported by others is crucial for adults as well; social support isn't just for kids and teenagers. Engaging others in activities such as cooking together or taking walks with friends can support the promotion of a healthy lifestyle.

Among other advantages, maintaining or reducing weight depends on scheduling regular physical activity.150 minutes a week of moderate aerobic exercise or 75 minutes a week of intense aerobic exercise.

The maintenance of weight requires both aerobic activity and weight training. Weight training that works all of your main muscles at least twice a week is advised by the WHO in addition to your weekly aerobic exercise.

Stress can alter eating habits and increase desires for high-calorie foods by triggering a brain reaction. Obesity can develop as a result of consuming excessive amounts of high-calorie foods.

Sustaining excellent health requires keeping a healthy weight. A wise place to start is by making lifestyle changes that will help prevent obesity. Obesity can be avoided with even modest lifestyle adjustments, including eating more veggies and working out occasionally a week.

A dietitian or simply nutritionist can give you the resources you'll require to get started if you're interested in taking a more individualized approach to your diet.

Finding the exercises that are most beneficial to your body can also be facilitated by scheduling a consultation with a fitness instructor or fitness teacher.

CHAPTER SIX; USING DIET TO REDUCE OBESITY.

By adhering to fundamental healthy eating guidelines, obesity can be avoided. Here are some easy dietary adjustments you may make to help you avoid obesity and lose weight.Consume five a day. Aim to consume between five and seven portions of total fruits and vegetables each day. Fruits and vegetables are foods low in calories. It is well supported by research that consuming fruits and vegetables lowers the risk of obesity. They are linked to a lower incidence of diabetes as well as insulin resistance, and they have higher nutritional contents. For example, its high fiber content makes you feel full on fewer calories, which helps you avoid gaining weight.Do not eat manufactured food. Empty calories are frequently found in highly processed meals like white bread as well as many packed snack foods, and they add up quickly.Cut back on sugar. It's critical to limit your consumption of added sugars. Avoid sugary drinks (such as sodas, energy drinks, and sports drinks); grain desserts (such as pies, cookies, and cakes); fruit juices (which are rarely made entirely of fruit juice); candies; and dairy desserts (such as ice cream).Cut back on artificial sweeteners. Obesity and diabetes have been associated with artificial sweeteners.

If you feel that you must add a sweetener, consider using a tiny quantity of honey as a healthier substitute.Instead, give attention to foods such as fruit such as avocados, olive oil, and tree nuts that are rich in healthy fats (polyunsaturated and monounsaturated fats). Even healthy fats should only make up 20% or 35% of daily calories; those who have high blood pressure or cardiovascular disease may require even lower amounts.Sip sensibly: Increase your water intake and cut out any sugar-filled drinks from your diet. Consider water your preferred beverage; coffee and tea without sugar are acceptable as well. Steer clear of energy drinks in general and sports drinks, as the former have been demonstrated to potentially harm the cardiovascular system in addition to having an excessive quantity of added sugar.Cook at home; those who do so are less likely to gain weight, regardless of gender. Additionally, they had a lower risk of type 2 diabetes.Give a plant-based diet a try. Consuming a diet composed of plants has been linked to a significantly decreased incidence of obesity and improved general health. At every meal, aim to fill your meal with whole fruits and vegetables. Eat tiny portions of unsalted nuts as a snack, such as pistachios, almonds, cashews, and walnuts—all of which are linked to heart health. Steer clear of protein

sources high in unhealthy fats, such
as dairy and red meat, or cut them out
completely.

Overweight individuals may benefit
from medical nutrition therapy. Those
with specific medical issues are also
eligible for it. A certified dietician will
collaborate with you during treatment
to create a personalized dietary plan.
A particular kind of healthcare
professional with expertise in nutrition
is a certified dietician. Their training
enables them to provide nutrition
counseling.

A dietitian will extensively examine
your eating habits throughout medical
nutrition therapy. Your new nutrition
objectives will be developed with his
or her assistance. Your nutritionist will
schedule multiple appointments with
you. After every appointment, he or
her will monitor your development.
You can create reasonable weight
loss objectives with the assistance of
your nutritionist. Approximately one to
one and a half pounds should be lost
per week by most people.

Medical nutrition therapy has been
shown to be beneficial for loosing
weight in many cases. To safely and
consistently reduce weight, a
nutritionist will advise you on the
number of calories you should
consume each day. You can plan a
wholesome, well-balanced diet with
their assistance. Making long-lasting,
healthy lifestyle adjustments can be
facilitated by this.

Even though a lot of people realize
they should reduce weight, many don't
know how. Your problems can be
addressed in collaboration with a

dietician. This is useful, according to
many.

It may go unnoticed by you that you
should consume more of some meals
while avoiding others. Alternatively, it's
possible that you already follow a
healthy diet but that you're consuming
too much. Changes that endure can
be achieved with the support of
medical nutrition therapy.

Those who have additional health
concerns can benefit from medical
nutrition therapy. In addition to those
who have undergone bariatric surgery,
this also covers those who suffer from
diabetes or cancer.

Chapter SEVEN; USING EXERCISE TO REDUCE OBESITY.

When you're attempting to lose
weight, boosting your level of physical
activity helps your body lose more
calories. By eating fewer calories
overall and burning fat through
physical activity, you can create a
calorie deficit and reduce weight. A
great deal of weight loss is attributable
to calorie restriction.

If a person wants to reduce weight,
they might need to combine food
changes with exercise. This should
include strength and aerobic exercise
as well.

Even while it is well established that
aerobic activity burns calories,
strength training preserves or helps

retain muscle when an individual loses weight in other areas.

Exercise can improve over time. several aspects for wellness from a trustworthy source Having stated that, everyone has different needs when it pertains to working out.

People who are novice to exercising should speak with a doctor beforehand to make sure their program is appropriate for them. In general, it is suggested that:

Take it slow at first: even a modest fitness regimen can significantly lower the potential danger of cardiovascular disease. Even if a person cannot manage to exercise for longer lengths of time, even up to ten minutes can be useful.

Modify your motions. Avoid taking on tasks that are too difficult for you. Instead, they can adjust their behavior based on how fit they are. For example, walking on flat ground or at a slower pace could be easier than sprinting or walking uphill. These adaptations allow one to push oneself farther as one gets fitter.

Consider lower-impact exercise: Yoga, water aerobics, and strolling on soft surfaces are some examples of activities that may ease strain on the body for people who experience joint soreness or related disorders.

Make movement a part of your daily routine. Physical activities include walking ascending and descending stairs, performing duties cultivating gardens, and playing with pets or children.

Consider signing up for a class. Exercise in a team can increase motivation, impart safety tips for certain activities, and give someone access to the expertise of a fitness teacher.

Consider physical treatment. A skilled therapist's individualized therapy may be helpful for someone who hasn't exercised recently or has chronic discomfort.

It could be advantageous for people who are new to it.

Should start with simpler workout routines, such as: Sit or stand with the arms out to the sides, rotating your trunk. With just your upper body, turn your trunk and arms to the side.

Sit-to-stand: Take a position near the edge of a firm, armless chair. As you rise up, take a breath, then release it again. After the subsequent exhale, gently realign your position.

Arm circles: Whether you're seated or standing, raise the arms to the sides. Keeping your arms straight, use your hands to draw small to large circles.

Arm raises: When standing or sitting, lift your arms straight in front of you and then gradually lower them back. People can lift both hands to the top end or sides of their heads.

Marching or stepping: Go for a short walk outside, stand on a small stool, or march in place.

By altering the repetitions, speed, or intensity of these workouts, one can tailor them to meet their own demands.

Many of the above-mentioned beginner exercises can be performed at home. For those seeking more energy, consider trying:

Stair climbing is a great aerobic and strengthening activity, particularly for the legs. People can walk or run while climbing and descending stairs. Bodyweight workouts are those that use an individual's own body weight as opposed to weights in order to develop muscles and bones. Leg lifts, squats, and lunges are a few examples.

Similar to tai chi and yoga, these exercises also employ your body weight and focus on flexibility, balance, and concentration. Someone may view free tutorial videos on the internet.

dance: Online resources offer a vast array of free dance fitness videos in various styles and skill levels.

There isn't any fitness workout that works for everyone. When creating a workout schedule that supports an individual in achieving their goals, factors such as their degree of fitness, general wellness, and personal preferences are taken into consideration.

Exercise should be challenging, but it shouldn't be cruel or agonizing. It could be entertaining or empowering. Over time, it can progressively improve a number of aspects of health.

If someone doesn't know where to begin or is having problems exercising, they might wish to see a doctor or physical therapist. Alternatively, individuals can experiment with different exercise routines by visiting by attending courses or using free online tools.

CHAPTER EIGHT; HOW LONG CAN WE CONTROL OBESITY.

You may lose weight on a diet plan more quickly the first week and then more gradually and steadily the next. Usually, during the first week, you lose a mix of water weight and body fat.
If this is the first time you have altered your eating and exercise regimen, weight reduction may happen more quickly. A weekly weight loss of 0.5-2 pounds is a reasonable goal to pursue.
Long-term results can be supported by a safe and sustained weekly weight loss of one to two pounds.
How can one lose weight the quickest?
You can achieve rapid and long-lasting weight loss by cutting back on calories and increasing your physical activity. Nevertheless, as every individual is unique, there can be another.
Age, gender, and beginning point are some of the variables that can impact the duration it takes you to shed weight. The duration may also be influenced by the ratio of calories you burn to calories you consume.
Losing some weight is a popular objective, whether it's for an important event or just to get healthier.
Perhaps you would like to understand what a suitable reduction in weight

rate is in order to set reasonable expectations.

You can read this book to learn more about the variables that influence how long weight loss may take.

You maintain your current weight if the amount of calories you take in and burn off is equal.

You need to produce a negative calorie balance—either by eating less than you burn off or by increasing your activity level—if you want to lose weight.

Although losing weight rapidly is what most people aspire to, it's crucial to avoid losing too much too soon. Dehydration, malnourishment, and gallstones can all be made worse by rapid weight loss.

Eating less than your energy expenditure leads to weight loss. Gender, age, initial weight, amount of sleep, and degree of calorie deficit are just a few of the many variables that impact how quickly you lose weight.

You might be curious how to gauge the time it may take you to attain your weight loss target if you're currently on one. Predicting with any degree of accuracy how long weight loss will take is generally impossible. The duration of weight loss is influenced by numerous factors. What you want to lose weight is a big factor.

The sort of weight you lose may also be predicted by your rate of weight loss. Losing more than two pounds each week for a few weeks is considered rapid weight loss.Two It has been demonstrated that progressive weight loss, as opposed to quick weight loss, results in the removal of more pounds of total fat and a lower body fat percentage—the body's ratio of fat weight to lean weight.

Many people can realistically lose a pound or two each week; drastic diet or exercise regimens shouldn't be necessary. But, because a higher calorie deficit may be produced by altering your diet, you might lose weight more quickly if you need to lose more weight.

How much time does weight loss take? It could be challenging to have reasonable expectations in this day and age of quick gratification and questionable marketing claims. Not to mention that you could be tempted to make yourself an aggressive weight loss target when you don't feel good about yourself and your wellness seems to be declining.

CHAPTER NINE; MAINTAINING THE WEIGHT LOSS.

Techniques for maintaining weight loss

Staying physically active is crucial for sustaining weight loss. Research indicates that even mild activity, like using the stairs and walking, has health benefits. It is advised to engage in weekly exercise that burns 1,500–2,000 calories in order to sustain weight loss.

Many people find it tough to lose weight, but maintaining their weight loss is even more difficult. The majority of people who lose a significant amount of weight gain it back two to three years later. One theory about weight gain is that individuals who reduce their caloric intake in an attempt to lose weight see a decline in the rate at which their physiques burn calories. As a result, losing weight becomes more challenging over several months. It can also be simpler to put on weight after a more regular diet is resumed if there is a decreased rate of calorie burning. These reasons make quick weight loss and extremely low-calorie diets undesirable.

It is advised to lose no more than half to two pounds every week. Making long-term lifestyle adjustments is necessary to improve the likelihood of long-term weight loss that is successful.

A person's health may improve if they lose weight to a healthy level for their height. These include reduced blood pressure, triglyceride and glucose levels, bone and joint stress, and cardiac workload. In order to reap the long-term health benefits of weight loss, maintenance is essential.

The following tactics that promote weight loss are crucial for maintenance as well:

Effective usage of support systems during weight loss can help maintain weight loss.

The National Weight Control Registry reports that 55% of registered members lost weight by following a program.

Staying physically active is crucial for sustaining weight loss. Research indicates that even mild activity, like using the stairs and walking, has health benefits. It is advised to engage in weekly exercise that burns 1,500–2,000 calories in order to sustain weight loss. Adults should aim to engage in moderate-to-intense physical activity for at least 40 minutes, three or four times a week. Exercise and diet are essential components of weight-loss and maintenance programs. In the National Weight Management Registry, 94 percent of registrants reported increasing their physical activity.

After achieving the target weight, a one-week trial of gradually increasing daily consumption of nutritious, low-fat meals by 200 calories may be conducted to observe whether weight loss persists. If losing weight does not stop, more calories from nutritious foods may be included every day until the ideal calorie balance for maintaining the target weight is found. Determining the effects of modifying food consumption and exercise intensity on weight may require some time and record-keeping. For this, a dietitian can be helpful.

Losing and gaining weight repeatedly is known as weight cycling. According to some research, "yo-yo dieting," or weight cycling, carries certain health hazards. Among them are hypertension, gallbladder disease, and hypercholesterolemia. These findings, however, do not apply to all people. Avoiding weight cycling and maintaining a healthy weight by making a commitment to more exercise and a balanced diet is the best course of action.

One misconception concerning weight cycling is that someone who loses and then gains weight will find it harder to maintain their new weight and lose it again than someone who has never experienced a weight-loss cycle. The majority of research indicates that riding weights has little effect on the body's fuel burning rate. Furthermore, the capacity to lose weight again is unaffected by a prior weight cycle. Furthermore, weight cycling has no effect on the distribution of fat around the stomach or the quantity of fat tissue.

DISCLAIMER.

The reader is not receiving specialized guidance or services from the publisher or author. The concepts, recommendations, and methods in the manuscript are not meant to replace consulting a professional.